Radical Fasting

DAVE WILLIAMS

Radical Fasting

Your Triple Benefits Rediscovered

DAVE WILLIAMS

Radical Fasting
Your Triple Benefits Rediscovered

ISBN 0-938020-69-2

First Printing 2002

Published by

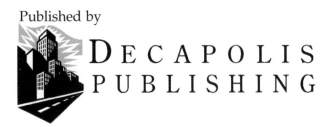

DECAPOLIS
PUBLISHING

Printed in the United States of America

BOOKS BY DAVE WILLIAMS

ABCs of Success & Happiness
The AIDS Plague
Angels: They are Watching You
The Art of Pacesetting Leadership
The Beauty of Holiness
The Christian Job Hunter's Handbook
The Desires of Your Heart
Depression, Cave of Torment
Developing the Spirit of a Conqueror
Filled: With the Mightiest Power in the Universe
Genuine Prosperity, The Power To Get Wealth
Getting To Know Your Heavenly Father
Gifts That Shape Your Life and Change Your World
The Grand Finale Revival
Grief and Mourning
Growing Up in Our Father's Family
Have You Heard From the Lord Lately?
How to Be a High Performance Believer
The Jezebel Spirit
The Laying on of Hands
Lonely in the Midst of a Crowd
Miracle Results of Fasting
The New Life . . . The Start of Something Wonderful
The Pastor's Minute
The Pastor's Pay
Patient Determination
Regaining Your Spiritual Momentum
Remedy for Worry and Tension
The Road To Radical Riches
The Secret of Power With God
Seven Signposts on the Road to Spiritual Maturity
Slain in the Spirit — Real or Fake?
Somebody Out There Needs You
Success Principles from the Lips of Jesus
Supernatural Soulwinning
Understanding Spiritual Gifts
What to Do If You Miss the Rapture
The World Beyond — The Mysteries of Heaven
Your Pastor: A Key to Your Personal Wealth

Contents

God is calling people to fast again, and not just to fast but to win souls.

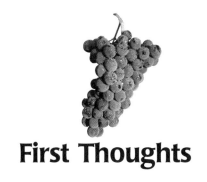

First Thoughts

What if I could show you something that would bring radical blessings to your life? Something that would cost you nothing and be harmless to others. Something that would:

• guarantee your success in getting rid of bad habits.

• help you to receive revelations from God.

• speed answers to prayer.

• rejuvenate your health.

• give you longer life.

• help you lose weight.

• slow the aging process.

• eliminate allergies.

• increase your energy level.

- give you mental clarity.

- break demonic forces.

- give you spiritual power.

This amazing practice is something I rediscovered just a few years ago, but already it has made a world of difference in my own life.

I'm talking, of course, about fasting—*Radical Fasting*. Fasting with purpose, precision, and power.

Perhaps you fast already, or maybe you fasted as a young Christian when you were just learning about the spiritual disciplines. Maybe you're like me and "forgot" the benefits of fasting for a while but now have a spiritual hunger that can't be satisfied any other way.

We live in one of those phenomenal seasons when God is calling people to fast again and not just to fast but to win souls, take spiritual authority seriously, and advance much faster in ministry than we ever have before. Underlying all these things is radical fasting which super-charges our efforts.

Radical fasting is not fasting longer or more often or with more extreme rules. I'm not proposing some sort of new legalism telling you to fast a certain number of days per month to achieve holiness. That's not what this is about.

Radical fasting is fasting effectively, confidently, with clear goals, knowing what the benefits are, and being determined to achieve them. It's:

- knowing that God will hear and answer,

- knowing what kind of attitude pleases the Lord in times of fasting, and what kind displeases Him,

- having a practical plan to guide you on your scheduled fast.

Are you ready to discover radical fasting and its powerful results?

Dave Williams

Lansing, Michigan

I had more revelation from God than I have ever had in my life.

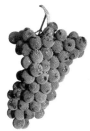

Chapter 1

How I Rediscovered Fasting

Nineteen-ninety-seven was one of those hard years for me. You know the kind. They seem to land like an elephant in your living room, taking up too much room, demanding all your time and energy, messing the place up, and refusing to leave.

It was one of those years when a lot of people I knew died. I conducted more funerals than in any other year of my ministry. I saw young men die leaving widows and children behind. I saw older men and women of God go to be with the Lord. I even saw teenagers and children snatched away before their time. After a while I considered dressing in my black suit all the time because I knew more funerals would be on the way.

I also struggled that year with the fact that Mount Hope Church had more than 6,000 people who called it their church home, but on any given Sunday morning we only saw about half of them. What were we doing wrong? Why weren't people coming to church more faithfully? What did that say about our effectiveness in growing mature Christian believers?

As a church, we were investing massive amounts of money and energy in evangelism efforts only to see things stay at roughly the same level. Why weren't we drawing more converts? Surely there were thousands who needed the Gospel in Lansing. For years our church had grown exponentially by winning souls and making disciples for our Lord. Had we lost our touch? Reached our limit? Run out of the blessing of the Lord?

I began crying out to God for some kind of breakthrough. I needed to punch a hole through the barriers that kept us from moving forward. I wanted to do battle, but none of my weapons seemed to work.

The Elusive Tape Set

I took a trip to a neighboring city to dedicate one of our daughter churches, and after the service I was in the foyer greeting people. I glanced over at the table where they were selling books and tapes and saw a tape album called, *Fasting for a Desired Result.* I hadn't seen that series before, and my heart leaped. I wanted to buy it, but by the time I got to the table, all the products had been packed away, and I decided not to bother anyone about it.

When I got home, I looked for it in our church bookstore and then in our warehouse. I couldn't find it anywhere. Still the idea of fasting or doing something — anything — to get a spiritual breakthrough was strong in my mind. That week one of my favorite evangelists, Dave Roever, visited our church, and as he and I were sitting in my office, I noticed that he had lost at least a hundred pounds. He seemed to have a new excitement and fervor for the ministry, and I asked him why. He said, "I fasted for forty days. Thirty days with nothing but distilled water and ten days with diluted juices. I had more revelation from God than I have ever had in my life."

Dave had been in the position I was in — desiring more from God and more out of his ministry — but unaware of how to break through. Finally, he turned to fasting, and the results were almost instantaneous. He began to hear God with more clarity. He lost all sorts of weight and took pressure off his heart. His ministry was imbued with an incredible power and effectiveness, so that souls were being won in great numbers. In every way, physically and spiritually, his life had improved.

God even told Dave what specific ministry goals to have. He told him to focus his efforts on Vietnam, that God was getting ready to bring in a great harvest there. Anyone who is familiar with Dave's ministry knows he had half of his face blown off in Vietnam when a sniper's bullet hit the grenade he was holding. He was not expected to live, but he pulled through with half his face scarred and deformed.

He had every reason to hate the Vietnamese, but God gave him a supernatural burden for the grandchildren of the people he fought in the war. He felt he needed to clothe and feed those children, but he didn't know where to get the money or how to make inroads in the tightly controlled Vietnamese government. After forty days of fasting, money started coming in to support the vision. He developed a relationship with a high-ranking official in Vietnam who gave him access to the permits and people needed to run a ministry there. Then the Japanese government called Dave and said, "We had an earthquake, and people from around the world donated clothes for children, but we have too much. We'd like to donate 1.1 million dollars worth of clothing to your ministry."

God advanced his ministry light years as a result of that forty-day fast, and people around the world were blessed!

I was so excited that I wanted to start fasting immediately, but I also wanted some teaching on the subject to make sure I was doing it effectively. Anyone who has fasted knows that it's best to go in with guidelines in place and to have access to encouragement in the form of testimonies or stories that build your faith, so you don't lose heart. I renewed my search for the fasting tape set I had seen, and finally someone on my staff found it. I popped the first cassette into my car stereo and began listening. The encouragement and teaching touched my heart, and I thought, "This is the most wonderful thing I've ever heard."

Then I realized it was my own sermon! I had forgotten that I preached on fasting eleven years earlier, and I barely recognized my own voice, but the truths coming through my car's speakers spoke deeply to me about this amazing practice. I was ready to rediscover radical fasting.

A Great Man Of Fasting And Faith

A few days later I attended a retirement banquet for Loren Triplett, the former Director of the Assemblies of God Foreign Missions ministry. I got to thinking about Loren. When he came to his post eight years earlier, the Assemblies had missionaries in eighty-six nations. By the time he retired, we had missionaries in one hundred and forty-eight nations. We had more growth in his term than in the whole history of our denomination. The number of people going to Assemblies of God churches around the world almost doubled.

All of us should be students of success, so I thought, "How did Loren do it? What made his work so effective?"

My mind went back to some of the things he talked about when we were together the three years I served on the missions board, and I realized that fasting was one of the cornerstones of his ministry. He always talked about how it was passed down to him from his parents who were early Pentecostal ministers. The more I thought about it the more sure I was that the secret of his achievements was his commitment to a fasted life.

For example, Loren and his wife, Millie, were young pastors when God told them, during a time of fasting, that He wanted them to be missionaries to Central America. Soon thereafter Loren spoke at a camp meeting and told of the instruction he had received. That night people laid money, diamond rings, and many other things of value at their feet. When they counted it all up it was enough to send them to the mission field right away. Typically it takes a missionary *eighteen months* to raise enough money to get to the field, but God did it in one night for the Tripletts.

The secret was fasting and prayer. They passed the practice on to their son, Don, who is today a missionary in Central America and one of the most effective men in our denomination. Sometimes he will find a mountain cave and fast a few days to seek the Lord. The Lord will give him revelation on what to do, where to go, and how to do it. This young man has reached 2.5 million people for Jesus Christ and has by far one of the largest missionary ministries in the world.

All of these thoughts came together for me after Loren's banquet when I had an extra day in Springfield, Missouri. I had planned to visit the Assemblies of God headquarters there and greet a few old friends, but as I got up that morning, the Holy Spirit was on me like a blanket, and I recognized that the day would hold something different. I couldn't get fasting out of my mind, so I sat down at the little desk in my hotel with nothing but a pencil and paper and wrote for twelve hours, producing the book *The Miracle Results of Fasting*.

I have never written a book in twelve hours. Some of the books I've written took me two years of hard work. It was the Holy Spirit moving my hand, enlightening my mind, touching my heart on this subject. I brought the scribbled-up paper back to my editorial staff and said, "Could you put this in book form by next week, so I can give everybody a free copy for our Christmas service?"

In seven days the book was edited and typeset with a terrific cover, and in a just a few weeks it was printed. Normally it takes at least ninety days to print a book, but we had it for the Christmas service, and I gave a copy to everyone who attended.

God not only wanted me to learn to fast, He wanted our whole church to be super-charged, radically fasting warriors because He has a purpose for us that requires added power and sensitivity to His voice.

I believe He has a purpose for you too. Can you think of an area of your life where you need a breakthrough? An area of your spiritual life that seems sluggish and resistant to change? Fasting may be just what you need! Read on to discover the amazing benefits of radical fasting.

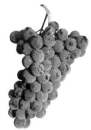

Chapter 2

The Triple Benefits Of Fasting

When you think of fasting, do you imagine someone with hollow cheeks, sunken eyes, and a somber demeanor?

Do you picture someone on a hunger strike to protest some global injustice?

Or do you picture someone who is vibrant, alive, with a new light in their eyes, and a bounce in their step?

That's really what fasting should produce. It's a biblical practice that has not one, not two, but three amazing benefits that happen to us all at once.

What is fasting? Simply put, it's abstaining from something, usually food, for a certain period of time. The word "fast" in Hebrew means to put your hand over your mouth. In Greek, it means to abstain from something, normally food.

The amazing thing about fasting is that it affects all three parts of our being. Paul said that each individual is made up of three parts: spirit, mind, and body. We are each a little trinity, a reflection of God. Most of the things we do in life affect only one or two parts of our being.

• Physical activity mainly helps our body and it also clears the mind.

• Education helps the mind but doesn't do much for the body or spirit.

• Worship is mainly a thing of the spirit though the Bible says to worship with our understanding and to demonstrate it with our bodies.

The practice of fasting seems to hit all three areas equally. It has triple benefits. It impacts all three parts of us in significant ways.

The first century church knew about the triple benefits of fasting. From time to time they called corporate fasts for specific purposes, and they also had regular times of personal fasting. One Bible dictionary said that early Christians fasted regularly on Wednesdays and Fridays, but after about a century, it became routine, and some were doing it to gain honor with men. So rather than temper the abuses with the proper use of this miraculous gateway to the supernatural, some of the church fathers discontinued it, and the power of fasting was lost.

Today people are realizing the triple benefits of fasting again and are reviving the practice. I have spoken with many believers who feel a personal conviction to start fasting regularly, and I know of many churches who embark on fasts together. I believe we have come full circle, and as the first century church practiced fasting, the end-time church is now practicing fasting.

Fasting In The Bible

Jesus fasted.

> After fasting forty days and forty nights, he was hungry.
>
> —Matthew 4:2

Jesus also endorsed fasting.

> When you fast, do not look somber as the hypocrites do ...
>
> —Matthew 6:16a

Notice He didn't say "if you fast" but "when you fast." Fasting was supposed to be a regular, healthy discipline of the Christian faith just like praying and reading the Bible.

Other great men and women of God fasted. In Luke, chapter two, we get a glimpse of a very old woman named Anna who spent her life in the temple fasting and worshiping. Some historical researchers say that she was between 106 and 110 years old! She was a prophetess and considered fasting and prayer her full-time ministry. We don't know if she fasted certain meals or if she fasted for days on end, but we do know fasting was such a prominent part of her ministry that the Holy Spirit forever enshrined it in His description of her in Luke's Gospel.

Anna's fasting led to one of the great moments in the Bible when she came to Mary and Joseph and prophesied over Jesus, who was an infant. Anna must have considered her years of fasting a small service compared to the honor God gave her of encouraging Jesus' parents and foretelling His ministry.

> **Coming up to them at that very moment, she gave thanks to God and spoke about the child to all who were looking forward to the redemption of Jerusalem.**
>
> **—Luke 2:38**

Anna became one of the first New Testament evangelists in the Bible!

Fasting was known even by non-Christians to be a powerful spiritual practice. Cornelius, a Roman centurion who didn't know Jesus yet, sought God through fasting and prayer with amazing results.

> And Cornelius said, Four days ago I was fasting until this hour; and at the ninth hour I prayed in my house, and, behold, a man stood before me in bright clothing, And said, Cornelius, thy prayer is heard, and thine alms are had in remembrance in the sight of God.
>
> —Acts 10:30-31 (KJV)

God sent Peter to Cornelius, and the whole household was saved. It became a major turning point when the church understood that God was pouring out His Spirit on non-Jews too. I can't help but notice that fasting brought the visitation to Cornelius. Maybe it was his way of showing God how earnest he was to know the truth.

Early Christians also used fasting as a way of learning God's will. In fact, Paul's ministry started during a season of fasting.

> In the church at Antioch there were prophets and teachers ... While they were worshiping the Lord and fasting, the Holy Spirit said, "Set apart for me Barnabas and Saul for the work to which I have called them." So after they had *fasted and prayed,* they placed their hands on them and sent them off.
>
> —Acts 13:1-3 (italics added)

Fasting was the normal practice the early Christians used to send out missionaries like Paul and

Barnabas, but it was also how they chose local church leaders. When Paul and Barnabas were in Galatia, they demonstrated this.

> Paul and Barnabas appointed elders for them in each church and, *with prayer and fasting,* committed them to the Lord, in whom they had put their trust.
>
> —Acts 14:23 (italics added)

Perhaps you feel like your ministry has never moved forward. Or maybe you haven't had the clarity of mind and spirit to recognize what He is telling you to do.

Have you had trouble finding your place in the local church? Have you bounced from one thing to another without settling down? Maybe God wants to kick-start your ministry during a time of fasting.

When you invest in yourself by fasting, you receive triple returns for your spirit, mind, and body. You'll never get that kind of yield in the stock market! Look more closely at what fasting can do for you.

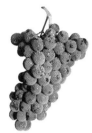

Chapter 3

Fasting For Health

Many people are surprised to learn that fasting is a healthy thing to do. It cleanses our bodies and helps us to achieve the natural balance that can be lost through modern diets and medicines.

My great grandfather was in his eighties when he was diagnosed with cancer. The surgeons told him that unless he had surgery he would die within a few months. He decided not to have the surgery but went back to his farm and started picking rhubarb and other vegetables and fruits out of the garden. He radically changed his diet and did away with meat and started boiling the rhubarb and vegetables for all his meals. (This was a Daniel fast which we will talk about later in the book.)

Not only did he live the rest of that year, he went on to live for sixteen more years and died not of cancer but because his heart finally gave out. Our bodies have been designed to heal themselves, and fasting allows that healing to take place. Hippocrates, the father of modern medicine, saw fasting as the remedy within. He said, "Everyone has a doctor in him or her, and we just have to help it in its work. The natural healing force within each one of us is the greatest force in getting well. Our food should be our medicine; our medicine should be our food but *to eat when you're sick is to feed your sickness*."

In other words, he recognized that our bodies are wired to fight sickness. He went on to say that if we are sick, it can be made worse if we keep feeding the sickness without a pause. That pause is fasting.

Fasting detoxifies our bodies. It removes toxic elements that come from the foods we eat. Look at the modern diet; it's full of artificial ingredients that our body was never intended to consume or absorb. Ice cream can contain formaldehyde to keep it from melting in the heat. Every kind of snack food, from potato chips to soda to gum contains artificial colors and flavors that are chemically produced and nondigestible. Even raw meats are treated with red dyes to give them a fresh look.

Vegetables and fruit can be full of pesticides, fungicides, herbicides, and insecticides that make the problem even worse — overburdening our delicate systems and eventually developing into disease. People are living longer these days, but they are also more diseased than ever. Heart disease, cancer, and a host of other ailments are caused or worsened by the stuff we consume. Without some way of detoxifying our bodies, we remain walking time bombs for disease.

Fasting helps eliminate these chemicals and poisons in our bodies. It gives our body a chance to fight back without having to constantly process new chemicals. Otto Buchinger, M.D., founded the famous Buchinger clinics in Europe that have had incredible success in curing people. Dr. Buchinger says that fasting is without a doubt "the most effective biological method of treatment." He calls it, "the operation without surgery" because it re-attunes, relaxes, and purifies our systems.

Buchinger has used fasting therapeutically for his patients, with astounding results. In fact, he has recorded results in curing cardiovascular and circulatory diseases, migraine headaches, glaucoma, digestive diseases, liver diseases, Crone's disease, chronic colitis, ulcerated colitis, degenerative diseases of the vertebral column, problems involving muscles and ligaments, skin diseases, allergies of the skin, cirrhosis, eczema, bronchial asthma, chronic sinusitis, and depression!

The Right Medicine

The advice given in the Bible almost always has a practical side to it, so I'm not surprised that fasting has been shown to be healthy. Why would God encourage a habit that was harmful? Isn't it like Him to add physical benefits to a spiritual discipline so that we receive more blessings?

There was a little boy named Jeff who at the age of eight started growing breasts. He didn't have any hair on his legs, and his genitals had never developed. His parents took him to a doctor, but a physical examination showed there was nothing wrong with him.

The doctor wasn't satisfied, so he researched toxicity and concluded that Jeff's body was not processing and eliminating estrogen, a female hormone. Something in his system was standing in the way. The doctor put him on a modified fast and detoxification program. In six weeks his breasts went down, hair appeared on his legs, and his genitals grew to the normal size for an eight-year-old.

Was the condition some freak genetic occurrence? No, he needed detoxification. He needed to fast.

I used to think that fasting was optional for a Christian, and certainly not something that encouraged health. Then I developed allergy problems and couldn't seem to overcome them. I was putting drops in my eyes to keep them from itching. I tried every medication on the market until finally I went to a Spirit-filled doctor, and he said, "Have you tried fasting?"

I reasoned, "Come on; don't you have a pill that can fix me?" He convinced me to try it, so I went on a fast, and the allergies subsided.

After that I noticed that certain foods would cause my allergies to flare up again. I would spread peanut butter on whole wheat bread and start sneezing. I would eat ice cream, and my eyes would start itching. I made a note of which foods caused problems, and I stopped eating them, and as a result I eliminated the wheezing, sneezing, and itching entirely. Fasting not only got me back on the right track, it helped me to identify problems in my diet. Then I began fasting those foods.

Dr. Joel Fuhrman in his book, *Fasting and Eating for Health*, said he believes that fasting and starting a natural diet should be the first treatment when someone discovers that she or he has a medical problem. He talks about research on animals at the New York

Academy of Science which showed that with periodic fasting, animal life spans increased up to twofold. Even animals benefit from fasting! If you love your dog or cat, make them fast one day a week and maybe they will live longer.

You will probably live longer, too, with regular fasting. This is brought out in the Bible. Remember that Anna the prophetess lived to be very old; so did many of the great men and women of God for whom fasting was a normal part of life.

Help To Conceive

Sylvia Franco was a medical doctor and had a master's degree in business by the time she was thirty years old. She kept in shape and ate properly, but she and her husband couldn't seem to conceive a child. She spent $100,000 on fertility doctors to no avail.

Finally she contacted a doctor who found that Sylvia was in some sort of toxic condition that was messing up her hormones. She had taken birth control pills for five years and several doses of an unusual type of antibiotic. Somehow it upset her balance. The doctor concluded that when she quit taking the birth control pills her hormone levels were all out of whack.

The doctor put her on a cleansing fast, and in three months she conceived a child.

Medicine can be a problem as well as a solution, if taken indiscriminately. At our church we found that the vast majority of people who come to us with problems of depression are taking medications that are not supposed to be taken together. Their problem seems to be the chemicals that mix or fight one another inside the body.

When my wife was pregnant, her doctor prescribed a pill for morning sickness. She asked about side effects, and he insisted there were none. When she inquired further, he became somewhat hostile and asked if she was questioning his integrity.

We didn't feel right about her taking the pills, so she refused to buy them and stopped seeing that doctor. We read a year later in the newspaper that those very pills can cause birth defects.

It's not wrong to take medicines, but we should think seriously about the ones we take. Putting chemicals into our bodies should not be as routine as some people make it out to be.

On the other hand, I have seen the value in taking natural supplements that get rid of the toxic chemicals in the body. I have felt so much better as a result! When Mary Jo and I were in London, England, we discovered that the exhaust was horrible in the downtown area. I had taken some Pycnogenol with us, which is an antioxidant that comes from a Mediterranean pine tree and is extremely powerful in fighting toxins. We took that before bedtime after walking around London all day, and in the morning we coughed and black stuff actually came out of our lungs! I can't imagine what that stuff would have done if left inside our bodies.

Fasting and taking antioxidants will help purify the body, but even if you don't take antioxidants, fasting alone will help your body achieve its natural balance. How much fasting you should do for physical benefit is up to you and your doctor. I recommend experimenting to see what you're able to do then doing it regularly. Your body will thank you!

Sometimes we need more than physical health. We need help or deliverance from a specific problem. That's the subject of our next chapter.

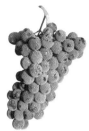

Chapter 4

Fasting For Help

Long-term health is good, but each of us knows what it's like to need fast solutions to a specific problem, whether it's financial, physical, or spiritual. Fasting is one of the best ways to get those solutions.

James Hammil was pastor of First Assembly of God in Memphis, Tennessee, and an executive presbyter for his denomination. One day he discovered he had cancer and was going to die. It was a heartbreaking discovery, especially since he didn't want to leave his church, and the church didn't want him to leave.

One of the elders went before the congregation and said, "Pastor's got cancer. The doctors say he's going to die. We can't afford to lose him. We need to fast." The church fasted on behalf of their pastor, and within a week, the cancer was gone. Hammil went on for many more years as pastor of that church.

Fasting brought a miracle of healing!

The Bible also shows us how judgment has been averted as a result of corporate fasting. The huge city of Ninevah, comparable in influence to New York City today, was marked for destruction, but when Jonah prophesied their destruction, the ruler of Ninevah called for a nationwide fast, and God gave them mercy instead.

Similar things have happened in our times. In the 1960s there was a great drought in America. Crops and livestock were dying, and farmers were suffering horribly. President Johnson called the nation to a time of fasting and prayer, and in three days the heavens broke open, the rain came down, and America was spared.

How Help Comes

Help can come in a variety of ways. First, God may grant or give you something in solution to your problem. It'll be like a UPS delivery truck pulling up to your house. You can fast when you need a financial miracle or breakthrough, and the solution will come in the form of a gift, something undeserved and unexpected. Many Christians, myself included, can

tell stories of receiving anonymous money or sur-
prise support in time of great need.

Secondly, God will deliver us from a problem or
deliver a foe into our hands. We all need deliverance
from certain habits or sins. In 2 Chronicles 20:3, King
Jehoshaphat and the nation needed deliverance from
three armies that were coming against Judah: Moab,
Ammon, and those on Mount Seir. Judah didn't have
a chance against them, so Jehoshaphat did the only
thing he knew might work: He called a fast.

That's when the deliverance began. For no appar-
ent reason, the enemy changed plans. Instead of at-
tacking Judah first, Moab and Ammon decided to
conquer Mount Seir first, so they slew all the people
on Mount Seir then said, "Now we can attack Judah."
But the Moabites began to suspect the Ammonites,
and the Ammonites began to distrust the Moabites,
and they went to war with each other until nobody
was left. Judah's enemies killed each other off, and it
all happened within three days of the time the nation started fasting and praying.

In the book of Esther, the Hebrew nation called a
fast, so they would not be wiped out by Haman's
evil plan, and a whole race of people was saved. It's
one of the most famous fasts in history.

That's the kind of power corporate fasting has.

Free From Demons

Thirdly, God will perform a supernatural feat to get you free, as when Jesus cast the demon out of a boy and said:

> ...this kind goes out not but by prayer and fasting.
>
> —Matthew 17:21 (KJV)

That boy was the recipient of supernatural deliverance that came not in the form of money or battlefield deliverance but a miracle of supernatural power.

I have friends named Liz and Fred who went through a terrible experience. Liz is a talented singer and had signed with a record company in New York to record Gospel music, but she discovered that people in the company were actually practicing witchcraft, mixing herbs, doing chants, and casting curses and hexes. Liz decided she didn't want to have anything to do with the company, so they decided to sue her for breach of contract.

Soon Liz became sick, and her daughter, Jasmine, began having unexplained seizures. Liz and Fred took Jasmine to the hospital. A brain scan showed that she had suffered twelve mini-strokes. There were five dark spots on her brain, eating it alive. She was dying by the minute, and doctors said she had only two days left.

When Liz saw the X-rays, God gave her a revelation that the devil was behind the attack. She took Jasmine home. They had to tie her to a wheelchair because the seizures would make her violent, and at times another voice would begin to speak through her saying things like, "I know about your sins, Liz." The voice even named sins from Liz's past; things her daughter didn't know anything about.

Not many Christians have faced spiritual warfare like this before. Until you come face to face with the devil, you don't know exactly what it's like. Liz had not been able to fast a day in her life before then, but her daughter was dying, and she urgently needed an answer, so she fasted for three days asking God to send someone to help her.

During this time of fasting, an old friend called and didn't know what Jasmine was going through. Liz explained the situation, and the friend recommended she go to a pastor that had a deliverance ministry. They took her to the service, and the pastor began to preach, but Liz grew more and more impatient, thinking, "My daughter's brain is under attack from the devil! Can't you start the prayer time?" But the Lord said, "Be still. Everybody has needs. You are going to be taken care of." Later in the service the pastor called Jasmine up and identified five demons that had taken control of her mind. He had not seen the X-rays and didn't know about the five dark spots. As he called them out one by one, Jasmine was delivered. Today she is a beautiful, vibrant young Christian lady with a touch of God on her life.

God worked supernaturally as a result of Liz's fasting. When we desperately need help, fasting is the best way to invite God's intervention. There will be many other wonderful examples throughout this book of God intervening as a result of fasting.

Fasting is also a wonderful tool for long-term spiritual growth, and we'll discuss that next.

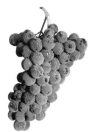

Chapter 5

Fasting For Holiness And Humility

Do you ever get into a routine where you're doing much more than you should, and it's wearing you down? It happens to me sometimes. My schedule turns around and latches onto me like a pit bull, and I feel gripped by urgency and stress.

Recently, when I was feeling that way, I plopped down on the floor and said, "God, I'm out of control. I need help to rein in my life, so it's manageable again." I felt the gentle nudge to fast, and it hit me again how easy the solution is, if only I would remember to do it.

Fasting does for us mentally what it does for us physically. It removes toxic thoughts from our minds. It humbles our soul and gives us a fresh poise. It makes us real before God. Through fasting we declare that God is more important and more essential than food or anything else that vies for our time. By fasting we fulfill the First Commandment, "You shall have no other gods before me" (Exodus 20:3). In fasting we say, "God You're my source. I'm accountable to You, and I'm going to show You that You're more important and more essential than my very life substance — food!"

These bodies of ours want to be number one. All day they whine, "I'm hungry. I want to look at this. I want to hear this. Feed me!" They get in the way of spiritual revelation, but fasting humbles them before God. David said:

> I humbled my soul with fasting.
>
> —Psalm 35:13b (KJV)

Every sincere Christian wants to be holier than he or she is. The Bible commands it, and our hearts desire it, though walking in holiness is often a struggle. Holiness means we deny what we want and embrace what God wants.

> If anyone would come after me, he must deny himself and take up his cross daily and follow me. For whoever wants to save his life will lose it, but whoever loses his life for me will save it. What good is it for a man to gain the whole world, and yet lose or forfeit his very self?
>
> —Luke 9:23-25

Fasting is a way of denying self and experiencing greater measures of holiness. Nothing makes us more real before God. Suddenly it becomes clear what is holy and what is unholy. You begin to see your heart for what it is, and it takes the pride right out of you!

In fasting, you have a deeper spiritual perception than ever before. Instead of constantly trying to impress other people, which is what most of us spend a good deal of time doing, you try only to impress God. That's why Jesus said, "When you fast be not as the hypocrites." Their fasting was an effort to impress men rather than God. True fasting brings humility that cares only what God thinks.

Mental Battles

Christians sometimes profess values that they don't really possess. They might profess peace but have conflict and are in terrible disarray because they run themselves ragged with an overloaded schedule. They might profess that family is important but don't slow down to enjoy their kids. They might profess to pray but rarely do it. Even Paul recognized this in himself.

> For what I do is not the good I want to do; no, the evil I do not want to do — this I keep on doing.
>
> **—Romans 7:19**

Like you and me, he was sometimes confused, sometimes in a mental battle. Whenever your mind is in a toxic state, not purified through fasting and reading the Word in prayer, the fleshly imagination will win over your will. When we fast, we put our spirit in charge of our minds. Jesus put it this way:

> The spirit is willing, but the body is weak.
>
> —Matthew 26:41b

Fasting puts the spirit in the driver's seat of our thoughts and actions so that we choose the holy things of God. This is what Paul meant when he wrote:

> Do not conform any longer to the pattern of this world, but be transformed by the renewing of your mind. Then you will be able to test and approve what God's will is — his good, pleasing and perfect will.
>
> —Romans 12:2

> ...I beat my body and make it my slave so that after I have preached to others, I myself will not be disqualified for the prize.
>
> —1 Corinthians 9:27

Fasting clears the mind and can even release us from mental disorders.

In a Moscow psychiatric unit, 7,000 patients had disorders ranging from schizophrenia to neurosis and had been treated with conventional medicine, but nothing seemed to help. The directors read Otto Buchinger's work and decided to try what they called the "hunger experiment." They quit feeding the patients for a week, giving them only water and sometimes juice. After that week, more than eighty percent of those patients were well enough to be released and live normal lives.

In Japan, the *Sapporo Medical Journal* reported that out of 382 patients with psychiatric diseases, eighty-seven percent were cured through the use of fasting. Somehow, fasting improves our ability to handle frustration and the stresses of life. God confirms this in His Word.

> You will keep in perfect peace, him whose mind is steadfast because he trusts in you.
>
> —Isaiah 26:3

The mental rewards of fasting are alone worth the price. We find a renewed closeness to God, a new power with God, and a greater sensitivity to spiritual things. The mind is clean, the body is being cleaned, and the search light comes on the soul to humble us. We may want to cry out like Isaiah did, "I am a man of unclean lips" (Isaiah 6:5), but we will surely find ourselves being drawn into a close relationship with God.

Now let's get on to some of the practical questions about fasting so we can succeed at it.

Fasts can differ from church to church and person to person.

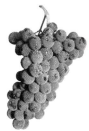

Chapter 6

Types Of Fasts

Have you encountered people who are proud about the way they fast or who look down their noses at people who don't fast as often as they do? Those kind turn fasting into a competition, but fasting is not a one-size-fits-all thing. The Bible tells about different kinds of fasts that were called for different purposes.

Fasts can differ from church to church and person to person. They even differ from situation to situation. There are two basic types of fasting: corporate fast and individual fast.

Corporate And Individual Fasting

A corporate fast is called by the leader of a nation, a tribe, a church, or a family. We have talked about King Jehoshaphat, the king of Ninevah, who called for a nationwide fast. There's power when a leader calls for a corporate fast. It's like a nation or church declaring war. I believe God magnifies their efforts more than we can possibly imagine.

Corporate fasts are also a time of detoxification for a church body. Impurities come to the surface where the Holy Spirit can blow them away, just as toxins are removed from our bodies. Until we fast, we don't know what impurities are there. When a church fasts together, they get to see each other in a much less polished way. Fasting can make you irritable, tired, and even mentally slow (temporarily, of course). It's easier to find fault with others and yourself.

This is part of the process. Let the Holy Ghost blow away those things like a cleansing breeze. Corporate fasts bring us to our knees together in repentance, and they draw us closer. We see each other for who we are (for better or worse!) and learn to love each other more deeply.

The second kind of fast is individual, when you declare a fast for personal reasons and don't wait for the pastor to declare a corporate fast. Both corporate and individual fasts greatly enhance our lives.

How To Fast

The most important rule of fasting to me is: *no legalism.* Fasting has no harsh rules or regulations. It's up to individual discretion how you fast. You can fast one day a week, two days a week, one day a month, two days a month, four times a year — whatever you feel the Lord is calling you to do. Once you settle on one way and feel it's the right one, *don't change it in the middle.* Stick with it! Abide by your commitment.

Sometimes I feel the need to fast for a week, sometimes for a day. Sometimes I fast all food, sometimes just meats and sweets. The Bible doesn't tell us exactly how to fast but shows a range of options.

> In weariness and painfulness, in watchings often, in hunger and thirst, in fastings often, in cold and nakedness.
>
> —2 Corinthians 11:27 (KJV)

Paul fasted often, but we don't know in what manner. If he was like the other New Testament believers, he probably fasted two days a week. I personally believe that Paul's fasts were short fasts. We have only one record where he was on a long fast, and that was probably for one week when he was on a ship in the middle of the storm.

> After the men had gone a long time without food...
>
> —Acts 27:21a

Clearly, if long fasts had been important to Paul, he would have made a point of recommending them.

The emphasis these days on fasting for forty days is perhaps a little overdone and might be keeping sincere people from trying to fast. First of all, fasting for forty days is hard on the body and the mind, and might not be right for everyone. Those leaders who have gone on forty-day fasts clearly had the Lord's leading. Others have tried only to find they couldn't go through with it, and after quitting in the middle felt like they had failed.

There are only two people for certain who fasted for forty days in the Bible, Jesus and Moses. Moses fasted when he was on the mountaintop receiving the Ten Commandments, and Jesus when He was being tempted in the desert.

Elijah may have fasted forty days. An angel came to him and gave him food from Heaven, and the Bible says that the food sustained him for forty days. It doesn't say that he fasted, but it's likely that he did. Interestingly, all three men appeared together when Jesus was transfigured before the disciples, with Moses representing the Law and Elijah the prophets.

There's no other record, in the entire Bible, of anybody fasting forty days on water alone. That's good news for those who aren't physically capable of fasting that long. The length of a fast is not important to

God. It isn't about winning a competition or going as long as you can. It's about humbling and chastening the soul. God is not measuring the length of time, but the sincerity of the heart.

Maybe you've been hung up by your inability to fast for a long time. Now is the time to let that go! God has given you freedom to choose a fast that fits you.

Daniel Fast

Fasting can also mean going without certain foods but not all foods. Some people fast two meals a day then have a very simple dinner (for example, a boiled potato and broth). Others eat normally but exclude meats and sweets. This is what the Bible describes as a "Daniel fast."

A "Daniel fast" refers to the prophet Daniel who was a palace assistant to the king of Babylon. When Daniel and his three friends were taken into captivity in Babylon, the king decided to train them for service. While living in the palace, Daniel saw that the king's table was spread out with steak, turkey, dressing, cranberry sauce, breads, pies, gravies, and all sorts of delicacies, but Daniel purposed in his heart not to eat of the king's delicacies. He didn't want to take part in the luxuries of Babylon or lose sight of God, so Daniel and his three friends ate nothing but vegetables (literally "pulce," that which came out of the earth). After ten days, the leader of the trainees looked at them and their complexion was fairer. They were healthier and more nourished than all the other ones that were eating at the king's table.

It goes on to say that Daniel became gifted in understanding visions and dreams and was considered ten times wiser than the others in the king's palace.

With the emphasis these days on lengthy or total fasts, I don't think some Christians realize the power of a Daniel fast. Daniel was given phenomenal gifts because of his faithfulness and fasting. God saw his heart not his plate. He realized that during a time of rigorous training, it was good to eat something, but that Daniel still made an effort to put God first.

A Daniel fast can be a powerful experience. We can gain just as much, or more, than on a total fast. It all depends on what we "purpose in our heart" to do. Is God leading you to go a week with only water? If so, He will provide the grace to carry it out. Is He asking you to go on a Daniel fast for a month? He'll give the grace for that too.

I often go on Daniel fasts and keep from eating pleasant foods, but if I need a little bit of energy to be in the pulpit on Sunday morning, I'll have a banana or a bowl of fruit with the other ministers before service. A Daniel fast is a good way to combat legalistic tendencies. It acknowledges that we need food but tells the soul that the only luxury we will enjoy during the fast is the luxury of God's presence.

Again, the important thing is to stick with the commitment you have made. Don't wake up each morning and decide what you will fast that day, and especially don't eat whenever you feel like it "in the name of grace." Fasting is a discipline. It's not supposed to be a strait jacket, but it doesn't mean we do whatever we want.

Getting the technical aspects of a fast right is important, but the spiritual aspects are much more important. Here are healthy things to do while you fast:

❑   Attend a prayer meeting at least once a week. If you're on a corporate fast, prayer meetings will become the heart of the church, as they should be anyway. Even if you're fasting individually, a prayer meeting will encourage you.

❑   Sign up as an intercessor. Maybe your church has backroom intercessors praying during each service. Put your prayer power to work when fasting.

❑   Read the Bible.

❑ Pray for your neighbors. Establish a "soul zone." Take daily walks around your neighborhood, and pray for each household as you pass by.

❑ Give up entertainment, television, radio, and videos for the duration of the fast.

❑ Do acts of kindness for people. Help a lady with her groceries, put a quarter in somebody's parking meter.

❑ Be a disciple maker.

When should you fast? That's the subject of the next chapter.

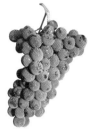

Chapter 7

When To Fast

We were having a corporate fast at my church one time when I heard a man say, "I think we're on this fast because Pastor Dave needed to go on a diet, and he didn't want to diet all by himself." Another lady wrote me and said, "You call Mount Hope the 'come as you are' church, but now you don't want fat people!"

Of course they were joking, but it's important to know when to fast. Seeing a few extra pounds register on the bathroom scale is not the best reason to fast, though losing weight is a nice side benefit (if you don't gain it all back later!).

How do we know when to fast? Do we wait for a sign from Heaven or a still, small voice in our spirit? I don't think so. If we wait for inspiration, we could be waiting a long time. Jesus simply said, "When you fast," not "When the Holy Spirit tells you to fast."

I don't usually feel inspired to fast, but I do it anyway. I don't always feel like praying or reading the Bible, but I do it anyway. The nature of discipline is that we don't always want to do the thing that is healthy for us.

What are some specific situations that should provoke you to fast?

When You're Facing A Mammoth Task

Nehemiah fasted before returning to Jerusalem to rebuild the wall. He needed the power and discernment to make right choices in what proved to be a massive undertaking.

Maybe you're facing such a task in your time. You might be:

- moving across the country.

- starting a business.

- establishing a new ministry.

- adopting children.

- facing new challenges at work.

Whenever you face a situation like Nehemiah's, where success will only come with God's help, that is a time to fast. You will see breakthroughs that once seemed unattainable.

When You're Facing Danger

> ...I proclaimed a fast, so that we might humble ourselves before our God and ask him for a safe journey for us and our children, with all our possessions.
>
> —Ezra 8:21

Sometimes we face physical danger. Maybe you're traveling to a foreign country. Maybe your son or daughter is serving in the military in a hot-spot or in war somewhere. I recently saw the parents of a young military man on the news. He was one of the crew on the spy plane that was detained in China for eleven days. In a television interview, this man's parents testified that they had sought the Lord for an answer to the crisis, and indeed, those service men and women were brought home without a scratch.

Maybe you're getting on an airplane in icy weather or going in for surgery. Any time we face danger is a good time to fast, even one meal or for a day.

When You Don't Know What To Do

We saw earlier how King Jehoshaphat called a national fast when he learned that his adversaries were marching against him (2 Chronicles 20). He didn't know what to do, and his first action was to fast.

When you don't know what to do, try fasting first. It works better than worrying or rushing around to force a solution. When you fast, you feel a sense of peace and rest knowing that you're doing everything you can, and that, ultimately, God will provide a solution.

When Your Nation Is Facing Moral Rot

Have you ever looked around you and been appalled at the society we live in? Has your spirit ever recoiled from what people think is acceptable entertainment? Acceptable morality? Acceptable business practices? Acceptable politics?

The prophet Joel saw his own nation in moral rot and said:

> **Declare a holy fast; call a sacred assembly.**
>
> **—Joel 1:14a**

When your heart is repulsed or grieved by what goes on in your nation, do the biblical thing, and fast. Not only will it call God's attention and invite His intervention, it will separate you and purify your own heart from unholy cultural influences.

When You Want To Change God's Mind

God doesn't change in character, but He will change His mind. He allows for true repentance to affect how He deals with people.

Jonah went to Ninevah and preached that God's judgment was falling on the city. The leader of the city called for a citywide fast.

> ...Do not let any man or beast, herd or flock, taste anything; do not let them eat or drink. But let man and beast be covered with sackcloth. Let everyone call urgently on God. Let them give up their evil ways and their violence. Who knows? God may yet relent and with compassion turn from his fierce anger so that we will not perish.
>
> —Jonah 3:7-9

God did change His mind and decided not to bring judgment on that city because they humbled themselves in fasting.

Maybe God's judgment is on you or your family because you have violated God's rules. Now is the time to fast. If you or someone you know has been in rebellion, repent from your ways, and then fast to show God you're serious about pleading for His mercy. You can change His mind!

When Commissioning Church Leaders

There are few things more important to a local church than choosing and commissioning leaders.

The men and women in charge will largely determine the course that church takes, whether to grow and prosper or stagnate and decline. Even if the entire congregation is ready to move forward, wrong leadership can thwart their efforts.

That's why every church should choose its leaders with the utmost care and spiritual discernment, and there's no better preparation than fasting. We saw earlier how the first-century church fasted and prayed before sending Saul and Barnabas off (Acts 13:2-3) and how Saul and Barnabas appointed elders in the churches only while fasting and praying. Should we do any less?

Whenever your church comes to a place of choosing its leaders, you should fast and pray that the right ones are chosen. This goes for all leadership positions, including nursery workers, musicians, even those who stand and greet people at the door. Every ministry is potentially life-changing to someone who visits for the first or hundredth time.

When You Feel Restless

Sometimes a creeping feeling of restlessness can come into your life, and sometimes it's God stirring you out of your comfort zone.

A friend of mine was pastoring a successful church. He had security, money, a nice car, and yet he felt restless. He fasted and prayed, and God said, "I want you to begin a home missions work in a totally different city." He left the security of that big church and went to a little town to begin a brand new work for God. He started a church with eleven other people, and today it's on course to having a broader influence than the church he left.

Sometimes that restless feeling is God moving you on. At other times it's not of God. The way to find out is to quiet yourself before Him with fasting and prayer. Your heightened spiritual perception will help you see which is the right way.

When Demonic Forces Are At Work In Someone's Life

Many Christians don't like to deal in the demonic realm (who would?), but it's part and parcel of the Gospel Jesus preached. We are told very plainly that some demonic strongholds will not be broken without fasting.

> And he [Jesus] said unto them, "This kind can come forth by nothing, but by prayer and fasting."
>
> —Mark 9:29 (KJV, brackets added)

Sometimes you can encounter problems that don't make any sense, except that a demon is causing them. When you suspect that this is true in your life or a friend's life, fast immediately. There's no reason to wait. Fasting gives us spiritual booster rockets to triumph over strong demonic oppression. Then you can pray and lay hands on that person with other Christians, and the bound-up person will be freed.

When Angelic Intervention Is Needed

We've all had times when we wished God would send angels to help us. The Bible says in a number of places that He does send angels. It's not our place to demand that God send angels, but we can acknowledge situations that require an extra measure of supernatural intervention.

The early church did this when Peter was put in prison. They had every reason to believe that King Herod would execute him. Stephen had already been stoned by an angry mob, and attacks of violence against believers were becoming common.

> ...but the church was earnestly praying to God for him [Peter].
>
> —Acts 12:5 (brackets added)

The night before Herod was to bring Peter to trial, an angel led him to safety through locked prison gates. Peter said:

> Now I know without a doubt that the Lord sent his angel and rescued me...
>
> —Acts 12:11

We are not told specifically that the church was fasting, but it's a good bet that they were. Fasting was such a normal practice of the church that Luke, the writer of Acts, might have simply assumed it. Or this might have been one of the church's regular times of fasting. In any case, God did send an angel to deliver Peter.

Daniel, the prophet, fasted and received an answer from Gabriel the archangel.

> ...Since the first day that you set your mind to gain understanding and to humble yourself before your God, your words were heard, and I have come in response to them.
>
> —Daniel 10:12

Can you imagine coming face to face with an angel? Daniel did and fell facedown, totally overwhelmed. He recognized that his situation was beyond his ability, and he fasted for supernatural intervention.

When A Friend Or Loved One Needs Our Prayers

Can we fast for others? Yes! Fasting is one of the most powerful things we can do on someone's behalf.

Most people have never heard of George McClosky. He was a man of God who had two daughters and one son. One day he decided that he was going to skip his lunch daily and spend that time praying for his children. In the course of time, his two girls married ministers, and the son went into the ministry. Pretty soon they started having children, and George decided to fast for his grandchildren too.

The grandchildren grew up and went to college. All of the girls married ministers and missionaries, and all of the boys went into the ministry or were preparing to go into the ministry except for one rebel who chose psychology, even though he felt guilty about it. He thought he was ruining a family tradition because everyone else had gone into the ministry, but his heart kept pulling him to psychology.

Did George's fasting and prayer work? Today that "rebel" has several best-selling books that help parents raise their children in a Christian way. He has one of the most popular Christian radio programs on the air. His name is Dr. James Dobson, and his career began with a fasting grandfather!

There are thousands of other reasons to fast, but these cover some of the basic ones. When should you fast? Whenever the Lord tells you, whenever your regular schedule tells you, or whenever you find yourself in a situation that demands extra spiritual power or assistance.

Your life will have spiritual booster rockets as a result!

We'll ask for His assistance, and immediately He'll say, "There you are."

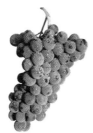

Chapter 8

The Rewards Of Fasting

Fasting isn't just about keeping ourselves from the pleasures of food. It's about gaining rewards. Is it biblical to fast for rewards? Absolutely! Jesus said:

> But when you fast, put oil on your head and wash your face, so that it will not be obvious to men that you are fasting, but only to your Father, who is unseen; and your Father, who sees what is done in secret, *will reward you.*
>
> —Matthew 6:17-18 (italics added)

The reward is the solution we seek, the answer we are hoping to gain, the provision, the deliverance, the comfort. I have not found a single fast in the Bible that didn't have a specific goal it was trying to achieve.

Is it okay to fast simply to draw close to God? Yes, but it's also healthy to fast with the expectation of receiving a specific answer. This does two things for us:

• It causes us to focus on the reward we seek not our hunger.

• It allows us to see God's faithfulness when the answer comes.

A terrible way to fast is to have: no reward ahead of you but the food you will eat when the fast is finished, every morsel of food you see look like a sirloin steak, and your appetite screaming so loud that you can't hear your own prayers.

When you fast for a reward, even the most succulent prime rib will look like cardboard compared to what you are expecting from God.

I know a man who fasted for his unsaved wife. One day she came to the church shaking like a leaf, ran to the altar, and accepted Christ. Over the years I have witnessed dozens of similar stories.

Determine The Reward

Write down what you need during a time of fasting. List your requests, and say, "Lord, these are the rewards that I want." Determine your reward before you enter the fast, and it will make fasting a joy.

The Bible's Rewards

The Bible is specific about some of the rewards we can expect when we fast. Isaiah 58 spells them out.

❑ *Reward #1: To loose the bands of wicked-ness.*

Bands are things that hold you back. It's what the writer of Hebrews meant when he wrote:

> ...let us throw off everything that hinders and the sin that so easily entangles, and let us run with perseverance the race marked out for us.
>
> —Hebrews 12:1

Have you ever known Christians who are held back? Nothing works for them? They plant seeds of faith, but the seeds don't grow? Perhaps they are held by bands of wickedness of their own doing. Only prayer and fasting can loose those bands so they can advance in the things of God.

❑ *Reward #2: To undo heavy burdens.*

The word "undo" means to violently shake off. Fasting doesn't just get rid of burdens that God never intended for us to carry; it violently shakes them off.

❑ *Reward #3: To let the oppressed go free.*

The discouraged, bruised, and wounded go free when we fast. The Hebrew word-picture here is of a vase that is cracking up. Have you ever felt like *you* were cracking up? That's a type of oppression. When you fast, you start a process of mending, becoming that beautiful vase God intended.

❏　***Reward #4: To break every yoke.***

A yoke is a bondage or a bad habit. When you fast, bad habits *will* be broken.

I used to have a bad coffee habit and was addicted to caffeine. I would drink three pots of coffee every day. Whenever I fasted I had terrible headaches. I thank God that I was delivered from caffeine in a matter of days by fasting. Now I can take it or leave it.

The same will happen to your bad habits. When the time of fasting ends, you can choose not to return to them.

❏　***Reward #5: Then your light will break forth as the morning.***

You will have revelation from God. Things will dawn on you. When I fast, the Bible comes alive to me, and I see things I never saw before. It's almost like revelations are spilling out faster than I can catch them.

Martin Luther translated the Bible from Hebrew and Greek to German, and he prayed and fasted over every word that he translated. That Bible is still being used by the German people today because Luther was guided by revelation.

❑ *Reward #6: Your health will spring forth speedily.*

We talked about health already. I knew a seventy-year-old man who had struggled with medical problems most of his life. He had been hospitalized many times, five times for asthma alone, and could find no relief until one doctor suggested that he go on an extended, supervised fast.

It was difficult at first. He seemed to be worse as he struggled to breathe, but he focused on the reward of good health. After six days, his enlarged prostate had shrunk to the size of a young man's. Then his sinuses cleared up. His breathing became normal, and on the thirty-sixth day, a miracle occurred when he regained permanent hearing in his deaf ear. A few days later he found that his sex drive had returned, and he was no longer impotent.

Talk about a bundle of rewards!

❑ *Reward #7: Your righteousness will go before you, and the glory of the Lord will be your rear guard.*

We all know the feeling of adversity, but this promise is that there will be no frontal attacks, and

God Himself will protect us from the things that come up behind us — the ones we don't see or expect.

❑   *Reward #8: Then you will call, and the Lord will answer.*

It's wonderful to have quick answers to prayer. During and after a fast, you will find that prayers are answered at lightning speed. You will pray, "Oh Lord, please ...," and the answer will zap you before you finish!

One time I was flying to Holland, and the Dutch stewardess seemed to know only one English phrase: "There you are." She helped me get my suitcase under the seat and said, "There you are." She walked by and filled my coffee cup and said, "There you are." No less than twenty-five times she said that to me.

Not only did I get a good laugh out of that, I got a picture of what God will do for us. We'll ask for His assistance, and immediately, with the provision delivered, He'll say, "There you are."

❑   *Reward #9: Then your light will rise in obscurity, and the darkness be as the noonday.*

The darkness that you have walked through is going to be broken, and your success will shine forth.

❏   *Reward #10: The Lord will guide you continually.*

Guidance can come in all sorts of ways. One time I was on vacation, and I heard about a certain up-and-coming company. As I was praying, God said, "Buy it!" So I called the church from the hotel and said, "Buy shares in this company." In less than a year, that stock had more than doubled, and we sold it.

I would like to be guided like that all the time!

❏   *Reward #11: The Lord will satisfy your soul in drought and make fat your bones.*

Once your health springs forth, God keeps you healthy through fasting. Not only that, but you will have a divine supply no matter what. You may get a pink slip on Monday, but you will know that God will provide. Fasting helps us to live not paycheck to paycheck but promise to promise. It helps us to see the reality of God's system that will never let the righteous go hungry.

❏   *Reward #12: Your children will build up the broken down places. You will be called the repairer of the breach, the restorer of paths to dwell in.*

God is going to use you to turn wastelands into fruitful orchards. Relationships that have gone sour can be restored with fasting. You will come into overflowing abundance.

Don't these sound like wonderful rewards? I know you have rewards you're seeking. Why not write them down, and plan a fast? You have nothing to lose (except a few pounds), and God will certainly show Himself faithful.

Next we'll look at a very specific reason to fast — when severe trouble hits.

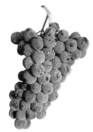

Chapter 9

Fasting To Drive Off Leviathan

This is a special chapter that applies to every Christian who has ever faced trouble. This chapter can save you months, even years, of heartache. It can help you through the most severe times of torment when you feel like you have become the special target of Hell.

The subject of this chapter is how to fast to drive off Leviathan. Who is Leviathan? He is a spiritual creature who ranks high in Satan's order of fallen angels.

Do such creatures exist? Paul said they did. He wrote:

> For we wrestle not against flesh and blood, but against principalities, against powers, against

> the rulers of the darkness of this world, against
> spiritual wickedness in high places.
>
> —Ephesians 6:12 (KJV)

Some of our most stubborn problems can be motivated by these evil powers.

- Insanity

- Persistent sin

- Depression

- Suicide thoughts

- Drug use

- Family and church division

Jesus cast a demon out of a boy who was rendered speechless and insane, and the boy returned to normal. Jesus cast demons out of the Gadarene man who lived among the tombs, cut himself with stones, and was incredibly violent. Jesus saw to the true problem not just the symptom, and the problem was demonic power.

Years ago, in the foyer of our old church, I was talking with a minister from a different church and he kept talking about Leviathan and how a prominent ministry had become caught in Leviathan's jaws. I didn't understand what he was talking about.

A year and a half later, I had my own encounter with Leviathan, though I didn't know what it was until later. I came to see that it was behind the problems that had come like an avalanche on me and the church.

What The Bible Says

I'm a preacher with fairly conservative beliefs. I don't go looking for exotic theories about the spirit world. But during this time of spiritual warfare, when our church was divided, I learned much about the dark, evil powers that work against believers.

Is Leviathan in the Bible? Yes, he is, but I didn't really pay attention until the bad circumstance rose over my head like a rushing river. During that time, I locked myself away in a Sunday school room for several hours a day and fought in the Spirit, and one day God gave me a vision. As I prayed I kept seeing a white, thick-skinned, crocodile-like creature. Finally I said, "Lord, what is that?" That's when the Lord first spoke to my heart and said, "Leviathan has been loosed against you."

I remembered the word "Leviathan" from the Bible, so I looked it up and found it first in Psalm 74:13-14.

> It was you who split open the sea by your power;
> you broke the heads of the monster in the wa-

> ters. It was you who crushed the heads of Levia-
> than and gave him as food to the creatures of
> the desert.

God began to reveal things about this creature that I had never considered. I had always thought it meant a sea creature or alligator of some kind, maybe one that had become extinct. I realized that the Psalm was not talking about a natural creature. The closest word we have in the English is crocodile or reptile, but God would never give reptile meat to His people to eat because that was considered unclean. There had to be a spiritual meaning.

I found the word again.

> In that day the LORD with his sore and great
> and strong sword shall punish leviathan the
> piercing serpent, even leviathan that crooked
> serpent; and he shall slay the dragon that *is* in
> the sea.
>
> —Isaiah 27:1 (KJV)

We all know there are no dragons in the sea. When prophets talk about the sea, it always means masses of people. In the book of Revelation, for example, it says the beast came out of the sea, meaning he came out of a group of people.

What did this verse in Isaiah tell me? That Levia-than was a spiritual creature important enough to mention in the Bible and important enough to show that one day the Lord would finish him off. The prophet called him a serpent, a term usually reserved for Satan himself. I concluded that he must be a powerful, hideous demonic creature who is apparently under the direct leadership of Satan himself and is assigned to bring down ministries, men and women of God, churches, families, and people who are seeking God.

The Crocodile

Next, I went to the encyclopedia to study crocodiles since that is the closest word-picture we get from the Hebrew translation. I learned that crocodiles always hang around water which is a symbol of God's Spirit and life. Jesus said:

> Whoever believes in me, as the Scripture has said, streams of living water will flow from within him.' By this He meant the Spirit ...
>
> —John 7:38-39a

Wherever the Holy Spirit is moving, you can be sure Leviathan is going to come.

Crocodiles put their eyes just above the water and look for a little duck, or a baby deer, or even a human being who comes up to the river to get a drink. We are supposed to be safe where the river of God is flowing, so Leviathan tries to make it unsafe. He wants us to close our spirits off because of fear. In one lightning leap, he will open his mouth and grab a victim in his jaws. His jaws are powerful enough to crush the victim, but the crocodile doesn't do that. He applies enough pressure to hold the victim in his mouth while he throws him back and forth until the victim becomes weary. Just when he thinks he might get free, the crocodile starts shaking him again until the victim loses all hope, and then the crocodile crushes and eats him.

Have you ever felt like you were being tossed back and forth with only brief moments of relief? That's the way Leviathan, the spiritual creature, works. He will try to whip you this way and that until you get so tired you become cynical and say, "What's the use?" and give up.

We don't need to succumb to him. We can recognize his character and defeat him.

His Character

How do we recognize Leviathan? What are his character traits? There are four.

❑   *Number One: He has many heads.*

The Psalmist spoke in the plural about the heads of the dragon. When there are many heads, there is confusion. One head says one thing, another head something else, and each head tries to speak with authority.

Families become this way when everyone thinks they are in charge. The instant result is confusion and distrust. Churches, too, are often afflicted by this multi-headed problem.

When Jesus was arrested, the witnesses couldn't get their stories straight. I believe Leviathan was loosed against Jesus causing confusion among the so-called witnesses.

Not only does he have many heads, but each claims to be right. When the Lord gave me a vision of Leviathan, I asked, "Why does he look like a white alligator?" The Lord said, "White is a symbol of righteousness. Leviathan always comes in the form of rightness and claims to be right."

Each head of Leviathan speaks to a different person, whispering in ears, convincing each that he or she is right. He works against our unity in the faith.

When unity starts to break down in relationships around you, you may be experiencing such an attack.

❑ *Number Two: He is piercing.*

The King James version calls him:

> ... the piercing serpent ...
>
> —Isaiah 27:1 (KJV)

The word "piercing" in Hebrew means roaming, shifting, focusing only on the temporary. Leviathan tries to get people to focus on the temporary rather than the eternal.

I have known people who roam from church to church within the same city. Their families are almost always unstable, and the children have trouble trusting Christians and rooting themselves in the Church.

Leviathan makes some wanderers, and they carry him everywhere they go. They reap no harvest except transience and confusion. A sense of rootlessness or an inability to connect at church can be a sign that you're under his attack.

❑   *Number Three: He seems bigger than he is.*

You know this feeling. Some problems seem oversized. Even prayer, it seems, can't send them away.

It's an interesting fact that most people who see crocodiles report them being thirty feet long, but the average crocodile only grows twelve to fifteen feet long. In other words, people think Leviathan is twice as big as he really is. Part of the devil's plan is to intimidate you into giving in so he won't have to fight. Nothing — not even Leviathan's attack — is ever as bad as it seems.

❑   *Number Four: He is crooked.*

Crooked means deceitful. A person who is affected by Leviathan will not give you a straight answer. You feel that you're dealing with something that you can't nail down.

The worst kinds of problems are those you can't identify. They are nebulous, like "the Blob" in the old horror movie. Leviathan doesn't walk in the front door and introduce himself. He is crooked, shifty, deceitful.

How To Get Rid Of Leviathan

How do we get rid of this horrible creature? There's only one way, and I know this from experience: fasting and prayer. Nothing else will do it, not good motives, not bright ideas, not friendly smiles, not emotional conversations, not meetings, not strategy, not quoting the Bible — nothing but the atomic bomb of fasting.

When God gave me the vision, I saw that the crocodile had thick skin. So I asked the Lord why, and He said, "Because you can throw rocks at him. You can hammer him. You can shoot at him with BB guns and pellet guns. You can yell at him. You can scream at him, but his skin is thick. It doesn't bother him at all." I said, "What do we do about him?" Immediately the

Scripture came to me, "This kind goeth forth not but by fasting and prayer."

I began fasting for a few days, and some who were closest to me joined in. Right before our eyes Leviathan started walking away.

I have studied revivals in my city of Lansing, and I discovered that no move of God has lasted more than four years. There have been sparks of revival in certain churches and ministries, but they haven't lasted long. Leviathan was trying to do to us what he had done for decades in Lansing, but we found the weapon he couldn't resist: fasting.

As soon as we started fasting, church attendance went up. Our church income began to soar. More people got saved than ever before.

Leviathan had one more trick before he disappeared. Remember that crocodiles have tails. When Leviathan is walking away from your family, home, church, ministry, or your business, he will take one last swipe at you with his tail. When he left our church, he swept a hundred people with him, and not partially committed people but good workers, board members, worship leaders, ushers, usher captains, teachers, children's ministers, and secretaries.

When he can't get you in his mouth, he swishes his tail in one final effort to bring you down, but with fasting and prayer, you can avoid the swishing tail of Leviathan.

I hope Leviathan is never loosed against you, but if he is, you know how to recognize him and drive him away: through fasting and prayer.

God responds to humility not an attitude that says, "I deserve a response."

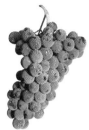

Chapter 10

Four Roadblocks To Effective Fasting

We have seen how fasting gives us good health and long life, how it invites God's supernatural intervention, and gives us keen spiritual perception.

We have seen how fasting moves us to deeper holiness, helps us to defeat Leviathan, and rescues us from mental confusion.

This chapter will show you four common roadblocks to effective fasting and how to remove them.

Is it possible to lose the rewards of fasting? Yes. Jesus warned of becoming a hypocrite because they fasted without any heavenly reward. There are four reasons our rewards will be rejected, and they all pertain to the attitudes of our heart.

❑   *Number One: Fasting to compete.*

> Your fasting ends in quarreling and strife, and
> in striking each other with wicked fists.
>
> —Isaiah 58:4a

Anyone who goes into a fast with a competitive spirit or thinking that it will show him to be holier than other people will lose the reward. If you're fasting everything but distilled water for ten days and you criticize someone else for doing a Daniel fast, you have lost your reward because your motivation is wrong. You are fasting with competitiveness.

If you're going to have a bad attitude or competitive spirit, call it a diet, not a fast!

It's also wrong to be silently competitive. If you delight in fasting because it makes you feel spiritually superior or worthy, that is just as wrong as making outright comparisons. Don't compete with others or with your own past "performance" in fasting, lest you lose your reward.

❑   *Number Two: Fasting in arrogance.*

Arrogance says, "I'm not going to eat until God does what I want." The point is to fast until God does what *He* wants. We have goals, but they had better be God's goals, or we are fasting in arrogance.

Years ago I found an old book on fasting and was encouraged to fast three days totally and then between sixty and ninety days on a Daniel fast. In that time I had more revelation from God than I had ever had. God spoke to me after the fast and said, "I have advanced your ministry by ten years."

That was not what I had fasted for. I didn't know exactly why I was fasting, but I knew I was being obedient to God, and He clearly had goals and purposes for me. My only purpose was to humble myself. I didn't stand up in arrogance and insist that God do something for me because I had discovered this spiritual discipline.

Less than two years later I became pastor of Mount Hope Church, though I was not even ordained. Some of the men in my own denomination didn't want me to pastor the church. I sat in one district meeting and slouched in my seat because they were discussing a resolution that said that only ordained Assembly of God ministers could pastor Assembly of God churches. I knew they were talking about me, but I didn't get angry or fight back. Instead I continued to lead the church as best I could, and that included regular times of individual and corporate fasting.

A few years later, after the church had grown from two hundred to seven hundred people, they decided to ordain me. We were seeing amazing miracles. Tumors would pop off people. One little girl was born without ears, and she got her hearing in one of our services. We fasted, and God caused the church to grow and prosper.

After a while, I became a hero to the men who had not wanted me to be pastor! I was given leadership positions on national committees and universities, *but not once did I fast to achieve any of it.* I never said, "God, I'm going to fast until You elevate me." I fasted for reasons that pleased God. My goals were His goals. I fasted not for personal gain but to advance His Kingdom. And I never fasted with an ultimatum that God had to do something. That's a hunger strike, not a fast.

I believe that the fasting I did as a young man laid the groundwork for my later ministry. Instead of reaching for the most prestigious things, I got on my face and humbled myself, and God opened doors that He saw fit to open. He responds to humility not an attitude that says, "I deserve a response."

❑ *Number Three: Fasting in a showy display.*

Remember, Jesus said:

> When you fast, do not look somber as the hypocrites do, for they disfigure their faces to show men they are fasting. I tell you the truth, they have received their reward in full. But when you fast, put oil on your head and wash your face, so that it will not be obvious to men that you are

fasting, but only to your Father, who is unseen; and your Father, who sees what is done in secret, will reward you.

—Matthew 6:16-18

When you enter a fast, don't make funny faces and proclaim what you're doing. The last thing you want is for people to say, "You are really spiritual" because then you will have received your entire reward.

A man invited me to lunch one time. He picked me up at the office and said, "By the way, I'm not eating today." I said, "But you invited me to lunch." He said, "I know, but I'm fasting!" If you're fasting, don't take people to lunch because it makes them feel guilty for eating, and they might think you're trying to "one-up" them.

Showy displays can also be subtle, as Jesus pointed out. You don't have to say anything, but if you put on a sad face or suck in your cheeks a little, you're accomplishing the same thing.

When fasting, act as normal as you can even if you feel weak or ill. Don't make your fasting the centerpiece of everyone else's life. Come out of the house smiling; go through your day like you do all other days. That way your reward will be secure.

❑   *Number Four: Fasting with boasting.*

Jesus gave the perfect example of this. Two men were praying. One said, "Lord, I sure thank You that I'm not like that sinner. I fast twice a week." The sinner said, "I'm a mess. God, be merciful to me." Jesus said the man who fasted twice a week went home unjustified, and the sinner who may not have fasted at all was justified in the sight of God! (See Luke 18:12.) That tells us that unless we get the heart attitude right, we may as well not fast.

Fasting in a showy display is like boasting to men, but when you start boasting to God, as this man did, you show just how backward your heart motivations are.

Fasting doesn't impress God. It never causes us to deserve anything. Everything depends on God's mercy. To boast to Him about our paltry efforts at righteousness is to give up our reward.

Once you remove these roadblocks to effective fasting you can move onto ways to super-charge your fast — the subject of the next chapter.

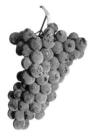

Chapter 11

Seven Tips To Super-Charge Your Fast

It's possible to go through a season of fasting feeling sluggish as if you're not advancing in the Spirit or hearing from God. Anyone who has tried fasting over the years probably knows the feeling.

Fasting doesn't need to be like driving in that old clunker that burns oil and always overheats. There are easy ways to turn your fast into a Lamborghini that is quick and responsive, making your season of fasting rewarding, fulfilling, encouraging, purifying, and exuberant. I call these the ways to super-charge your fast, and they are found in Nehemiah 9:1-3.

> On the twenty-fourth day of the same month, the Israelites gathered together, fasting and wearing sackcloth and having dust on their heads. Those of Israelite descent had separated themselves from all foreigners. They stood in

> their places and confessed their sins and the
> wickedness of their fathers. They stood where
> they were and read from the Book of the Law of
> the LORD their God for a quarter of the day,
> and spent another quarter in confession and in
> worshiping the LORD their God.

Let's look at the seven principles in this account.

❑   *Number One: Get together with other Christians.*

During times of corporate fasting the church needs to assemble more. The pastor needs to schedule extra prayer meetings so people are encouraged and feel they are part of a bigger cause.

I mentioned before that it's also important to go to prayer meetings if you're on an individual fast. You will appreciate the energy and anointing you receive to help you keep going.

It's even a good idea to meet with other Christians in your neighborhood. Whatever you do, stay plugged in with other believers.

❑   *Number Two: Get separated.*

The Israelites cut themselves off from any non-believing influence. This doesn't mean you should cut yourself off from co-workers, friends, or unsaved family, but that you deliberately, willfully purpose in your heart to focus on God and stay away from non-believing influences. This may mean a person, a television show, a radio program, certain magazines, the internet, or books.

Your spirit is especially open during a time of fasting. You are more sensitive not only to godly forces but to unclean forces. If you allow something in that is impure, it will have a deeper effect on you.

It's impossible to avoid going to work or driving down the street for the duration of a fast, but you can put a guard over your eyes and control your thoughts and mentally block things out that get in the way of what the Lord is doing.

❑   *Number Three: Confess your sins.*

Confession is like putting a gasoline additive into your tank to burn out the junk that builds up in the engine. The apostle John wrote:

> **If we confess our sins, he is faithful and just and will forgive us our sins and purify us from all unrighteousness.**
>
> —1 John 1:9

There's nothing better about fasting than the clean feeling it gives you in your spirit. During times of fasting, we see things in our lives that we need to confess. Name them specifically to the Lord. You will feel so free!

❑ *Number Four: Confess the sins of past generations.*

Why would we want to dig up the sins of our forefathers? Because there are some people that are saved but not delivered. There are people who love God but are in bondage. I believe that there are things called generational curses that are passed down.

Have you noticed how certain problems afflict certain families for generations? Heart trouble, anger, crime, drug use, obesity, and gluttony. These sins become generational curses that the devil uses to trip up each new batch of children.

We may not even know the sins of past generations, but we should confess that we come from a line of sinners and then, through the blood of Jesus, reverse that curse. Daniel, the prophet, did this. He laid himself out before the Lord and confessed the sins of his forefathers just as if he had committed the sins himself.

I believe that we can also confess the sins of our president, governors, and mayors. There's power in acknowledging sin, even if we didn't "do" the sin.

❑   *Number Five: Spend extra time in God's Word.*

> They stood where they were and read from the Book of the Law of the LORD their God...
>
>   —Nehemiah 9:3a

The people in Nehemiah's day gave themselves constant exposure to God's Word while they fasted.

If you want to super-charge your fast, spend more time in the Word. Listen to tapes of the Bible or preaching. Let your open spirit absorb all the rich nutrients of God's Word.

❑   *Number Six: Confess the Word of God.*

> ... and spent another quarter [of the day] in confession ...
>
>   —Nehemiah 9:3b (brackets added)

This is different than acknowledging sin. It's to confess what God says is true. It means verbally affirming the Word of God. For example, say, "I'm an overcomer by the blood of the Lamb and the word of my testimony." Or "I can do all things through Christ who strengthens me."

Speaking with faith like that will get you through the times when your body feels weak.

❏   *Number Seven: Worship.*

Worship is heart-to-heart communion with God. Jesus said true worshipers worship the Father in Spirit and truth. Never will your worship soar like when you're fasting! You will have confessed your sins, confessed your forefathers' sins, been filled of the Word, gathered with other believers, and put off anything that would contaminate your mind. That's a recipe for super-charged worship!

These seven tips will get you out of a rut and onto the road. They will put a 300-horsepower engine on your fasting times, and you will advance faster than you could have imagined.

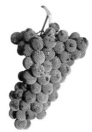

The Last Word

Fasting essentially does one thing: It places us in a position to receive from God. It doesn't earn His favor or get His attention. It doesn't produce faith, but it does put a razor's edge on the faith we already have.

Fasting intensifies God's power in our lives. My most rewarding memories come from times when I fasted and felt the nearness of God like never before.

Here are a few reminders of what we have learned in this book. Treat them like a checklist to make your next time of radical fasting a success.

❑ *Make a firm commitment to God and to yourself.*

❑ *Don't listen to your appetite. Remember what Paul said, and keep your body under subjection and present it as a living sacrifice.*

❑   *List the rewards you're expecting. Write them down, and review them daily in prayer.*

❑   *Pray extra during times of fasting.*

❑   *Give up secular television and secular videos.*

❑   *Select a plan for fasting, and stick to it.*

❑   *Stay focused on the benefits.*

May your life be enriched and blessed because of radical fasting!

About The Author

Dave Williams is pastor of Mount Hope Church and International Outreach Ministries, with world headquarters in Lansing, Michigan. He has served for over 20 years, leading the church in Lansing from 226 to over 4000 today. Dave sends trained ministers into unreached cities to establish disciple-making churches, and, as a result, today has "branch" churches in the United States, Philippines, and in Africa.

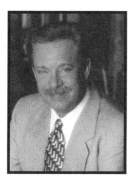

Dave is the founder and president of Mount Hope Bible Training Institute, a fully accredited institute for training ministers and lay people for the work of the ministry. He has authored 50 books including the eighteen-time best seller, *The New Life...The Start of Something Wonderful* (with over 2,000,000 books sold), and more recently, *The Miracle Results of Fasting*, and *The Road To Radical Riches*.

The Pacesetter's Path telecast is Dave's weekly television program seen over a syndicated network of secular stations, and nationally over the Sky Angel satellite system. Dave has produced over 125 audio cassette programs including the nationally acclaimed *School of Pacesetting Leadership* which is being used as a training program in churches around the United States, and in Bible Schools in South Africa and the Philippines. He is a popular speaker at conferences, seminars, and conventions. His speaking ministry has taken him across America, Africa, Europe, Asia, and other parts of the world.

Along with his wife, Mary Jo, Dave established The Dave and Mary Jo Williams Charitable Mission (Strategic Global Mission), a mission's ministry for providing scholarships to pioneer pastors and grants to inner-city children's ministries.

Dave's articles and reviews have appeared in national magazines such as *Advance, The Pentecostal Evangel, Ministries Today, The Lansing Magazine, The Detroit Free Press* and others. Dave, as a private pilot, flies for fun. He is married, has two grown children, and lives in Delta Township, Michigan.

You may write to Pastor Dave Williams:

P.O. Box 80825

Lansing, MI 48908-0825

Please include your special prayer requests when you write, or you may call the Mount Hope Global Prayer Center anytime: (517) 327-PRAY

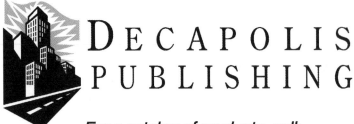

DECAPOLIS PUBLISHING

For a catalog of products, call:

1-517-321-2780 or

1-800-888-7284

or visit us on the web at:

www.mounthopechurch.org

For Your Spiritual Growth

Here's the help you need for your spiritual journey. These books will encourage you, and give you guidance as you seek to draw close to Jesus and learn of Him. Prepare yourself for fantastic growth!

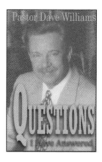

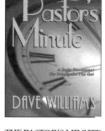

QUESTIONS I HAVE ANSWERED
Get answers to many of the questions you've always wanted to ask a pastor!

THE PASTOR'S MINUTE
A daily devotional for people on the go! Powerful topics will help you grow even when you're in a hurry.

ANGELS: THEY'RE WATCHING YOU!
The Bible tells more than you might think about these powerful beings.

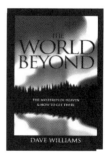

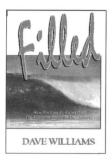

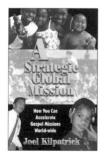

THE WORLD BEYOND
What will Heaven be like? What happens there? Will we see relatives who have gone before us? Who *REALLY* goes to Heaven?

FILLED!
Learn how you can be filled with the mightiest power in the universe. Find out what could be missing from your life.

STRATEGIC GLOBAL MISSION
Read touching stories about God's plan for accelerating the Gospel globally through reaching children and training pastors.

These and other books available from Dave Williams and:

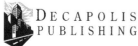

DECAPOLIS PUBLISHING

For Your Spiritual Growth

Here's the help you need for your spiritual journey. These books will encourage you, and give you guidance as you seek to draw close to Jesus and learn of Him. Prepare yourself for fantastic growth!

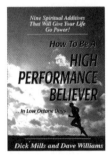

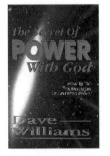

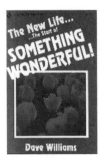

HOW TO BE A HIGH PERFORMANCE BELIEVER
Pour in the nine spiritual additives for real power in your Christian life.

THE SECRET OF POWER WITH GOD
Tap into the real power with God; the power of prayer. It will change your life!

THE NEW LIFE ...
You can get off to a great start on your exciting life with Jesus! Prepare for something wonderful.

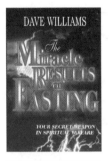

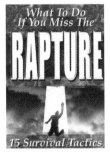

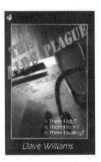

MIRACLE RESULTS OF FASTING
You can receive MIRACLE benefits, spiritually and physically, with this practical Christian discipline.

WHAT TO DO IF YOU MISS THE RAPTURE
If you miss the Rapture, there may still be hope, but you need to follow these clear survival tactics.

THE AIDS PLAGUE
Is there hope? Yes, but only Jesus can bring a total and lasting cure to AIDS.

These and other books available from Dave Williams and:

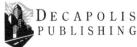
DECAPOLIS PUBLISHING

For Your Spiritual Growth

Here's the help you need for your spiritual journey. These books will encourage you, and give you guidance as you seek to draw close to Jesus and learn of Him. Prepare yourself for fantastic growth!

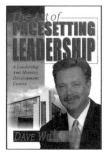

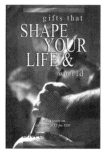

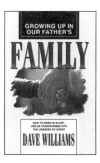

THE ART OF PACESETTING LEADERSHIP
You can become a successful leader with this proven leadership development course.

GIFTS THAT SHAPE YOUR LIFE
Learn which ministry best fits you, and discover your God-given personality gifts, as well as the gifts of others.

GROWING UP IN OUR FATHER'S FAMILY
You can have a family relationship with your heavenly father. Learn how God cares for you.

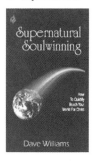

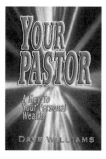

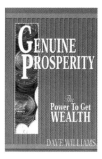

SUPERNATURAL SOULWINNING
How will we reach our family, friends, and neighbors in this short time before Christ's return?

YOUR PASTOR: A KEY TO YOUR PERSONAL WEALTH
By honoring your pastor you can actually be setting yourself up for a financial blessing from God!

GENUINE PROSPERITY
Learn what it means to be truly prosperous! God gives us the power to get wealth!

These and other books available from Dave Williams and:

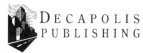

D E C A P O L I S
P U B L I S H I N G

For Your Spiritual Growth

Here's the help you need for your spiritual journey. These books will encourage you, and give you guidance as you seek to draw close to Jesus and learn of Him. Prepare yourself for fantastic growth!

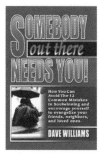

SOMEBODY OUT THERE NEEDS YOU
Along with the gift of salvation comes the great privilege of spreading the gospel of Jesus Christ.

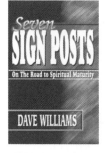

SEVEN SIGNPOSTS TO SPIRITUAL MATURITY
Examine your life to see where you are on the road to spiritual maturity.

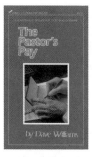

THE PASTORS PAY
How much is your pastor worth? Who should set his pay? Discover the scriptural guidelines for paying your pastor.

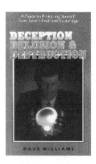

DECEPTION, DELUSION & DESTRUCTION
Recognize spiritual deception and unmask spiritual blindness.

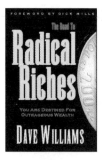

THE ROAD TO RADICAL RICHES
Are you ready to jump from "barely getting by" to Gods plan for putting you on the road to Radical Riches?

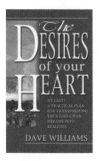

THE DESIRES OF YOUR HEART
Yes, Jesus wants to give you the desires of your heart, and make them realities.

These and other books available from Dave Williams and:

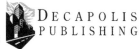

For Your Successful Life

These video cassettes will give you successful principles to apply to your whole life. Each a different topic, and each a fantastic teaching of how living by God's Word can give you total success!

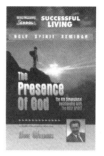

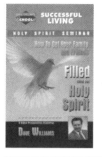

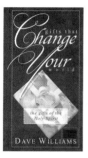

THE PRESENCE OF GOD
Find out how you can have a more dynamic relationship with the Holy Spirit.

FILLED WITH THE HOLY SPIRIT
You can rejoice and share with others in this wonderful experience of God.

GIFTS THAT CHANGE YOUR WORLD
Learn which ministry best fits you, and discover your God-given personality gifts, as well as the gifts of others.

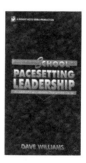

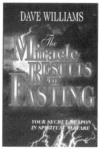

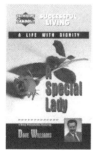

THE SCHOOL OF PACESETTING LEADERSHIP
Leaders are made, not born. You can become a successful leader with this proven leadership development course.

MIRACLE RESULTS OF FASTING
Fasting is your secret weapon in spiritual warfare. Learn how you'll benefit spiritually and physically! Six video messages.

A SPECIAL LADY
If you feel used and abused, this video will show you how you really are in the eyes of Jesus. You are special!

These and other videos available from Dave Williams and:

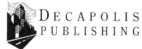

DECAPOLIS PUBLISHING

For Your Successful Life

These video cassettes will give you successful principles to apply to your whole life. Each a different topic, and each a fantastic teaching of how living by God's Word can give you total success!

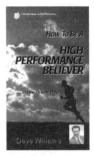

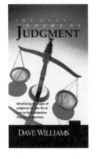

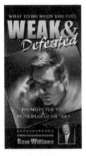

HOW TO BE A HIGH PERFORMANCE BELIEVER
Pour in the nine spiritual additives for real power in your Christian life.

THE UGLY WORMS OF JUDGMENT
Recognizing the decay of judgment in your life is your first step back into God's fullness.

WHAT TO DO WHEN YOU FEEL WEAK AND DEFEATED
Learn about God's plan to bring you out of defeat and into His principles of victory!

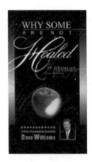

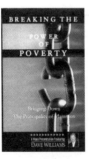

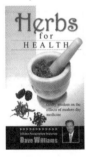

WHY SOME ARE NOT HEALED
Discover the obstacles that hold people back from receiving their miracle and how God can help them receive the very best!

BREAKING THE POWER OF POVERTY
The principality of mammon will try to keep you in poverty. Put God FIRST and watch Him bring you into a wealthy place.

HERBS FOR HEALTH
A look at the concerns and fears of modern medicine. Learn the correct ways to open the doors to your healing.

These and other videos available from Dave Williams and:

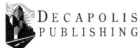

DECAPOLIS PUBLISHING

Expanding Your Faith

These exciting audio teaching series will help you to grow and mature in your walk with Christ. Get ready for amazing new adventures in faith!

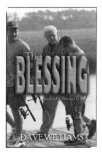

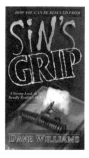

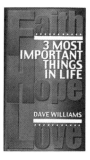

THE BLESSING
Explore the many ways that God can use you to bless others, and how He can correct the missed blessing.

SIN'S GRIP
Learn how you can avoid the vice-like grip of sin and it's fatal enticements that hold people captive.

FAITH, HOPE, & LOVE
Listen and let these three "most important things in life" change you.

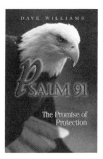

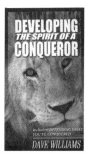

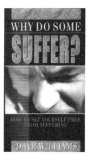

**PSALM 91
THE PROMISE OF
PROTECTION**
Everyone is looking for protection in these perilous times. God promises protection for those who rest in Him.

**DEVELOPING
THE SPIRIT OF A
CONQUEROR**
You can be a conqueror through Christ! Also, find out how to *keep* those things that you have conquered.

WHY DO SOME SUFFER
Find out why some people seem to have suffering in their lives, and find out how to avoid it in your life.

These and other audio tapes available from Dave Williams and:

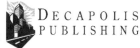

DECAPOLIS PUBLISHING

Expanding Your Faith

These exciting audio teaching series will help you to grow and mature in your walk with Christ. Get ready for amazing new adventures in faith!

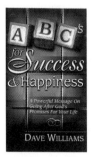

ABCs OF SUCCESS AND HAPPINESS
Learn how to go after God's promises for your life. Happiness and success can be yours today!

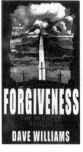

FORGIVENESS
The miracle remedy for many of life's problems is found in this basic key for living.

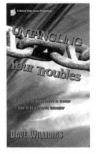

UNTANGLING YOUR TROUBLES
You can be a "trouble untangler" with the help of Jesus!

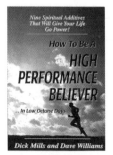

HOW TO BE A HIGH PERFORMANCE BELIEVER
Put in the nine spiritual additives to help run your race and get the prize!

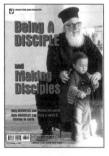

BEING A DISCIPLE AND MAKING DISCIPLES
You can learn to be a "disciple maker" to almost anyone.

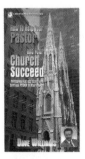

HOW TO HELP YOUR PASTOR & CHURCH SUCCEED
You can be an integral part of your church's & pastor's success.

These and other audio tapes available from Dave Williams and:

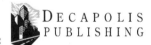

DECAPOLIS PUBLISHING

For other products by Dave Williams check out are website at: **www.mounthopechurch.org**